The Super Tasty Ketogenic Diet Recipe Collection

A Complete Guide to Boost Your Metabolism with Delicious Recipes

AF256284

Michelle Lewis

1

© Copyright 2021 - All rights reserved.

The content contained within this book may not be reproduced, duplicated or transmitted without direct written permission from the author or the publisher.

Under no circumstances will any blame or legal responsibility be held against the publisher, or author, for any damages, reparation, or monetary loss due to the information contained within this book. Either directly or indirectly.

Legal Notice:

This book is copyright protected. This book is only for personal use. You cannot amend, distribute, sell, use, quote or paraphrase any part, or the content within this book, without the consent of the author or publisher.

Disclaimer Notice:

Please note the information contained within this document is for educational and entertainment purposes only. All effort has been executed to present accurate, up to date, and reliable, complete information. No warranties of any kind are declared or implied. Readers acknowledge that the author is not engaging in the rendering of legal, financial, medical or professional advice. The content within this book has been derived from various sources. Please consult a licensed professional before attempting any techniques outlined in this book.

By reading this document, the reader agrees that under no circumstances is the author responsible for any losses, direct or indirect, which are incurred as a result of the use of information contained within this document, including, but not limited to, — errors, omissions, or inaccuracies.

Contents

Chicken Bacon Soup 7

Cream Pepper Soup 10

Ham Asparagus Soup 13

Beef Zoodle Soup 16

Broccoli Cheese Soup 18

Italian Stuffed Mushrooms 21

One-Pot Mushroom Stroganoff 23

Avocado with Pine Nuts 25

Zucchini Noodles with Famous Cashew Parmesan 26

Cream of Broccoli Soup 28

Swiss Chard Chips with Avocado Dip 30

Banana Blueberry Smoothie 32

Cajun Artichoke with Tofu 33

Mushroom and Cauliflower Medley 35

Spicy and Peppery Fried Tofu 37

Colorful Creamy Soup 39

Tofu Stuffed Zucchini 41

Broccoli Masala 43

Italian-Style Tomato Crisps 45

Lebanese Asparagus with Baba Ghanoush 47

Garlic Mozzarella Bread 49

Truffle Parmesan Bread 51

Truffle Parmesan Salad 54

Cashew Siam Salad... 56

Avocado and Cauliflower Hummus... 58

Raw Zoodles with Avocado and Nuts.. 60

Cauliflower Sushi 63

Spinach and Mashed   Tofu Salad...66

Ketogenic Curry Almond Bread 69

Egg Roll Bowl 71

Shio Koji Karaage Tofu 73

Zoodle Pesto Salad 75

Cucumber Edamame Salad...77

Flourless Bread 79

Walnut & Mushroom Loaf..82

Maple Low Carb Oatmeal...85

Easy Curried Tofu Scramble...87

Vegan Low Carb Superfood Bowl 90

Yogurt Parfait..92

Shirataki Noodles with Almond Butter Sauce 93

Chocolate Sea Salt Smoothie 95

Ingredient Zucchini Lasagna 96

Vegan Ketogenic Scramble 98

Low Carb Ramen...100

Low Carb Smoked Salmon Chowder..102

Ketogenic Bone Broth..104

Slow Cooker Vegetable Beef 106

Beef Cabbage...109

Ketogenic Chicken 111

Chicken Bacon Soup

Preparation Time: 10 minutes

Cooking Time: 40 minutes

Servings: 4

Ingredients:

6 boneless, skinless chicken thighs make cubes.

½ cup chopped celery.

4 minced garlic cloves

6-ounce mushrooms, sliced.

½ cup chopped onion.

8-ounce softened cream cheese

¼ cup softened butter

1 teaspoon dried thyme

Salt and (finely ground) black pepper, as per taste preference.

2 cups chopped spinach.

8 ounces cooked bacon slices, chopped.

3 cups (preferably homemade) chicken broth

1 cup heavy cream

Directions:

Arrange Instant Pot over a dry platform in your kitchen. Open its top lid and switch it on.

Add the ingredients except for the cream, spinach, and bacon; gently stir to mix well.

Close the lid to create a locked chamber; make sure that safety valve is in locking position.

Find and press "SOUP" cooking function; timer to 30 minutes with default "HIGH" pressure mode.

Allow the pressure to build to cook the ingredients.

After cooking time is over press "CANCEL" setting, find and press "NPR" cooking function. This setting is for the natural release of inside pressure and it takes around 10 minutes to release pressure slowly.

Slowly open the lid, stir in cream and spinach.

Take out the cooked recipe in serving plates or serving bowls and enjoy the Ketogenic recipe. Top with the bacon.

Nutrition:

Calories: 490.

Carbohydrates: 7g.

Protein: 23g.

Fat: 6g.

Sugar: 2.2g.

Sodium: 742mg.

Fiber: 1.7g

Cream Pepper Soup

Preparation Time: 8-10 minutes

Cooking Time: 10 minutes

Servings: 4

Ingredients:

1 (preferably medium size) celery stalk, chopped.

1 (preferably medium size) yellow bell pepper, chopped.

1 (preferably medium size) green bell pepper, chopped.

2 large red bell peppers, chopped.

1 small red onion, chopped.

2 tablespoons butter

1/2 cup cream cheese, full fat

1/4 teaspoon dried thyme, (finely ground)

1/2 teaspoon black pepper, (finely ground)

1 teaspoon dried parsley, (finely ground)

1 teaspoon salt

2 cups vegetable stock

1 cup heavy cream

Directions:

Arrange Instant Pot over a dry platform in your kitchen. Open its top lid and switch it on.

Find and press "SAUTE" cooking function; add the butter in it and allow it to heat.

In the pot, add the onions, bell pepper, and celery; cook (while stirring) until turns translucent and softened for around 3-4 minutes.

Pour in the vegetable stock and heavy cream — season with salt, pepper, parsley, and thyme.

Close the lid to create a locked chamber; make sure that safety valve is in locking position.

Find and press "MANUAL" cooking function; timer to 6 minutes with default "HIGH" pressure mode.

Allow the pressure to build to cook the ingredients.

After cooking time is over press "CANCEL" setting, find and press "QPR" cooking function. This setting is for quick release of inside pressure.

Slowly open the lid, mix in the cream; take out the cooked recipe in serving plates or serving bowls, and enjoy the Ketogenic recipe.

Nutrition:

Calories: 286.

Carbohydrates: 9g.

Protein: 4g.

Fat: 0g.

Sugar: 2g.

Sodium: 445mg.

Fiber: 0g

Ham Asparagus Soup

Preparation Time: 10 minutes

Cooking Time: 55 minutes

Servings: 4

Ingredients:

5 crushed garlic cloves

1 cup chopped ham.

4 cups (preferably homemade) chicken broth

2 pounds trimmed and halved asparagus spears.

2 tablespoons butter

1 chopped yellow onion.

½ teaspoon dried thyme

Salt and freshly (finely ground) black pepper, as per taste preference.

Directions:

Arrange Instant Pot over a dry platform in your kitchen. Open its top lid and switch it on.

Find and press "SAUTE" cooking function; add the butter in it and allow it to heat.

In the pot, add the onions; cook (while stirring) until turns translucent and softened for around 4-5 minutes.

Add the garlic, ham bone and broth; stir, and cook for about 2-3 minutes.

Add the other ingredients; gently stir to mix well.

Close the lid to create a locked chamber; make sure that safety valve is in locking position.

Find and press "SOUP" cooking function; timer to 45 minutes with default "HIGH" pressure mode.

Allow the pressure to build to cook the ingredients.

After cooking time is over press "CANCEL" setting, find and press "QPR" cooking function. This setting is for quick release of inside pressure.

Slowly open the lid, add the prepared recipe mix in a blender or processor.

Blend or process to make a smooth mix. Place the mix in serving bowls and enjoy the Ketogenic recipe.

Nutrition:

Calories: 146.

Carbohydrates: 5g.

Protein: 29.4g.

Fat: 6g.

Sugar: 2.2g.

Sodium: 222mg.

Fiber: 4g

Beef Zoodle Soup

Preparation Time: 5 minutes

Cooking Time: 13 minutes

Servings: 4

Ingredients:

4 tablespoons Avocado oil

3 tablespoons Minced ginger

1 tablespoon Minced garlic

1 ½ pound Sirloin steak tips, cut into 1-inch pieces.

2 cups Broccoli florets

8 ounces Bella mushrooms, sliced.

6 cups Beef broth

1/4 cup Apple cider vinegar

1/4 cup Coconut aminos

1/4 cup Sriracha sauce

1 large zucchini, spiralized into noodles

Directions:

Switch on the instant pot, grease pot with oil, press the 'sauté/simmer' button, wait until the oil is hot and add the steak pieces along with ginger and garlic.

Cook steak for 5 minutes or more until nicely golden brown, then add remaining ingredients except for zucchini and stir until mixed.

Press the 'keep warm' button, shut the instant pot with its lid in the sealed position, then press the 'manual' button, press '+/-' to set the cooking time to 8 minutes and cook at high-pressure setting; when the pressure builds in the pot, the cooking timer will start.

When the instant pot buzzes, press the 'keep warm' button, do a quick pressure release and open the lid.

Taste the soup to adjust seasoning, add zucchini noodles and toss until just mixed.

Ladle the soup into bowls and serve.

Nutrition:

Calories: 239.

Carbohydrates: 3g.

Protein: 29g.

Fat: 11g.

Sugar: 5g.

Sodium: 254mg.

Fiber: 1g

Broccoli Cheese Soup

Preparation Time: 10 minutes

Cooking Time: 12 minutes

Servings: 5

Ingredients:

2 tablespoons Butter, unsalted

2 tablespoons Minced garlic

3 cups Vegetable broth

6-ounce Broccoli florets

1 cup Monterey jack cheese, shredded.

2 cups, and 2 tablespoons Sharp cheddar cheese, shredded.

1 tablespoon Dijon mustard

½ teaspoon Paprika

⅛ Teaspoon Ground black pepper

1 cup Heavy whipping cream

¼ teaspoon Salt

1 teaspoon Xanthan gum

Directions:

Switch on the instant pot, add butter, press the 'sauté/simmer' button, wait until the butter melts, and add garlic and cook for 1 minute or until fragrant.

Stir in broth, cook for 1 minute, then add broccoli florets and stir until mixed.

Press the 'keep warm' button, shut the instant pot with its lid in the sealed position, then press the 'manual' button, press '+/-' to set the cooking time to 10 minutes and cook at high-pressure setting; when the pressure builds in the pot, the cooking timer will start.

When the instant pot buzzes, press the 'keep warm' button, do quick pressure release and open the lid.

Add mustard, Monterey jack cheese, and 2 cups of cheddar cheese, season with black pepper and paprika and stir until cheese begins to melt.

Then pour in the cream, stir until well-incorporated and taste to adjust salt.

Take out ¾ cup of soup, add xanthan gum, stir well, then add into the soup in the instant pot and stir well until well combined.

Garnish soup with remaining cheddar cheese and serve.

Nutrition:

Calories: 276.

Carbohydrates: 5.1g.

Protein: 11.8g; Fat: 23.8g.

Sugar: 2.2g; Sodium: 509mg.

Fiber: 0g

Italian Stuffed Mushrooms

Preparation Time: 10 minutes

Cooking Time: 35 minutes

Servings: 4

Ingredients:

- 1-pound button mushrooms, stems removed
- 2 tablespoons coconut oil, melted
- 1-pound broccoli florets
- 1 Italian pepper, chopped
- 1 teaspoon Italian herb mix
- Salt and pepper, to taste
- 1 shallot, finely chopped
- 2 garlic cloves, minced
- 1 cup vegan parmesan

Directions:

1. Parboil the broccoli in a large pot of salted water until crisp-tender, about 6 minutes. Mash the broccoli florets with a potato masher.

2. In a saucepan, melt the coconut oil over a moderately-high heat. Once hot, cook the shallot, garlic, and pepper until tender and fragrant. Season with the spices and add in the broccoli.

3. Fill the mushroom cups with the broccoli mixture and bake in the preheated oven at 365 degrees F for about 10 minutes.

4. Top with the vegan parmesan and bake for 10 minutes more or until it melts.

Nutrition:

206 Calories

13.4g Fat

12.7g Protein

4g Fiber

One-Pot Mushroom Stroganoff

Preparation Time: 10 minutes

Cooking Time: 25 minutes

Serving: 4

Ingredients:

- 2 tablespoons canola oil
- 1 parsnip, chopped
- 1 cup fresh brown mushrooms, sliced
- 1 cup onions, chopped
- 2 garlic cloves, pressed
- 1/2 cup celery rib, chopped
- 1 teaspoon Hungarian paprika
- 3 ½ cups roasted vegetable broth
- 1 cup tomato puree
- 1 tablespoon flaxseed meal
- 2 tablespoons sherry wine
- 1 rosemary sprig, chopped
- 1/2 teaspoon dried basil
- 1/2 teaspoon dried oregano

Directions:

1. In a heavy-bottomed pot, heat the oil over a moderately-high flame. Cook the onion and garlic for 2 minutes or until tender and aromatic.

2. Add in the celery, parsnip, and mushrooms, and continue to cook until they've softened; reserve.

3. Add in the sherry wine to deglaze the bottom of your pot. Add in the seasonings, vegetable broth, and tomato puree.

4. Continue to simmer, partially covered, for 15 to 18 minutes. Add in the flaxseed meal and stir until the sauce has thickened.

Nutrition:

114 Calories

7.3g Fat

2.1g Protein

3.1g Fiber

Avocado with Pine Nuts

Preparation Time: 5 minutes

Cooking Time: 10 minutes

Serving: 4

Ingredients:

- 2 avocados, pitted and halved
- 1 tablespoon coconut aminos
- 1/2 teaspoon garlic, minced
- 1 teaspoon fresh lime juice
- Salt and pepper, to taste
- 5 ounces pine nuts, ground
- 1 celery stalk, chopped

Directions:

1. Thoroughly combine the avocado pulp with the pine nuts, celery, garlic, fresh lime juice, and coconut aminos. Season with salt and pepper to taste.
2. Spoon the filling into the avocado halves.

Nutrition:

263 Calories

24.8g Fat

3.5g Protein

6.1g Fiber

Zucchini Noodles with Famous Cashew Parmesan

Preparation Time: 5 minutes

Cooking Time: 15 minutes

Serving: 4

Ingredients:

For Zoodles:

- 2 tablespoons canola oil
- 4 zucchinis, peeled and sliced into noodle-shape strands
- Salt and pepper, to taste

For Cashew Parmesan:

- 1/2 cup raw cashews
- 1/4 teaspoon onion powder
- 1 garlic clove, minced
- 2 tablespoons nutritional yeast
- Sea salt and pepper, to taste

Directions:

1. In a saucepan, heat the canola oil over medium heat; once hot, cook your zoodles for 1 minute or so, stirring frequently to ensure even cooking.
2. Season with salt and pepper to taste.

3. In your food processor, process all ingredients for the cashew parmesan. Toss the cashew parmesan with the zoodles and enjoy!

Nutrition:

145 Calories

10.6g Fat

5.5g Protein

1.6g Fiber

Cream of Broccoli Soup

Preparation Time: 5 minutes

Cooking Time: 15 minutes

Serving: 4

Ingredients:

- 1-pound broccoli, cut into small florets
- 8 ounces baby spinach
- 4 cups roasted vegetable broth
- 2 tablespoons olive oil
- 1 yellow onion, chopped
- 2 garlic cloves, minced
- 1/2 cup coconut milk
- Salt and pepper, to taste
- 2 tablespoons parsley, chopped

Directions:

1. Heat the oil in a soup pot over a moderately-high flame. Then, sauté the onion and garlic until they're tender and fragrant.
2. Add in the broccoli, spinach, and broth; bring to a rolling boil. Immediately turn the heat to a simmer.
3. Pour in the coconut milk, salt, pepper, and parsley; continue to simmer, partially covered, until cooked through.

4. Puree your soup with an immersion blender.

Nutrition:

252 Calories

20.3g Fat

8.1g Protein

4.5g Fiber

Swiss Chard Chips with Avocado Dip

Preparation Time: 10 minutes

Cooking Time: 20 minutes

Serving: 6

Ingredients:

- 1 tablespoon coconut oil
- Sea salt and pepper, to taste
- 2 cups Swiss chard, cleaned

Avocado Dip:

- 3 ripe avocados, pitted and mashed
- 2 garlic cloves, finely minced
- 2 tablespoons extra-virgin olive oil
- 2 teaspoons lemon juice
- Salt and pepper, to taste

Directions:

1. Toss the Swiss chard with the coconut oil, salt, and pepper.
2. Bake the Swiss chard leaves in the preheated oven at 310 degrees F for about 10 minutes until the edges brown but are not burnt.
3. Thoroughly combine the ingredients for the avocado dip.

Nutrition:

269 Calories

26.7g Fat

2.3g Protein

4.1g Fiber

Banana Blueberry Smoothie

Preparation Time: 5 minutes

Cooking Time: 0 minutes

Serving: 4

Ingredients:

- 1/2 cup fresh blueberries
- 1/2 banana, peeled and sliced
- 1/2 cup water
- 1 ½ cups coconut milk
- 1 tablespoon vegan protein powder, zero carbs

Directions:

1. Blend all ingredients until creamy and uniform.

Nutrition:

247 Calories

21.7g Fat

2.6g Protein

3g Fiber

Cajun Artichoke with Tofu

Preparation Time: 15 minutes

Cooking Time: 30 minutes

Serving: 4

Ingredients:

- 1-pound artichokes, trimmed and cut into pieces
- 2 tablespoons coconut oil, room temperature
- 1 block tofu, pressed and cubed
- 1 teaspoon fresh garlic, minced
- 1 teaspoon Cajun spice mix
- 1 Spanish pepper, chopped
- 1/4 cup vegetable broth
- Salt and pepper, to taste

Directions:

1. Parboil your artichokes in a pot of lightly salted water for 13 to 15 minutes or until they're crisp-tender; drain.
2. In a large saucepan, melt the coconut oil over medium-high heat; fry the tofu cubes for 5 to 6 minutes or until golden- brown.
3. Add in the garlic, Cajun spice mix, Spanish pepper, broth, salt, and pepper. Add in the

reserved artichokes and continue to cook until for 5 minutes more.

Nutrition:

138 Calories

8.9g Fat

6.4g Protein

5g Fiber

Mushroom and

35

Cauliflower Medley

Preparation Time: 15 minutes

Cooking Time: 30 minutes

Serving: 4

Ingredients:

- 8 ounces brown mushrooms, halved
- 1 head cauliflower, cut into florets
- 1/4 cup olive oil
- 1/2 teaspoon turmeric powder
- 1 teaspoon garlic, smashed
- 1 cup tomato, pureed
- Salt and pepper, to taste

Directions:

1. Toss all ingredients in a lightly oiled baking pan.
2. Roast the vegetable in the preheated oven at 380 degrees F for 25 to 30 minutes.

Nutrition:

113 Calories

6.7g Fat

5g Protein

2.7g Fiber

Spicy and Peppery Fried Tofu

Preparation Time: 10 minutes

Cooking Time: 20 minutes

Serving: 2

Ingredients:

- 2 bell peppers, deveined and sliced
- 1 chili pepper, deveined and sliced
- 1 ½ tablespoons almond meal
- Salt and pepper, to taste
- 1 teaspoon ginger-garlic paste
- 1 teaspoon onion powder
- 6 ounces extra-firm tofu, pressed and cubed
- 1/2 teaspoon ground bay leaf
- 1 tablespoon sesame oil

Directions:

1. Toss your tofu, with almond meal, salt, pepper, ginger-garlic paste, onion powder, ground bay leaf.
2. In a sauté pan, heat the sesame oil over medium-high heat.
3. Fry the tofu cubes along with the peppers for about 6 minutes.

Nutrition:

223 Calories

15.9g Fat

15.6g Protein

3.3g Fiber

Colorful Creamy Soup

Preparation Time: 10 minutes

Cooking Time: 25 minutes

Serving: 6

Ingredients:

- 2 cups Swiss chard, torn into pieces
- Sea salt and pepper, to taste
- 2 thyme sprigs, chopped
- 2 teaspoons sesame oil
- 1 onion, chopped
- 2 bay leaves
- 6 cups vegetable broth
- 1 cup grape tomatoes, chopped
- 1 cup almond milk, unflavored
- 1 teaspoon garlic, minced
- 2 celery stalks, chopped
- 1 zucchini, chopped
- 1/2 cup scallions, chopped

Directions:

1. In a heavy bottomed pot, heat the sesame oil in over a moderately-high heat. Sauté the onion, garlic, and celery, until they've softened.

2. Add in the zucchini, Swiss chard, salt, pepper, thyme, bay leaves, broth, and tomatoes; bring to a rapid boil. Turn the heat to a simmer.

3. Leave the lid slightly ajar and continue to simmer for about 13 minutes. Add in the almond milk and scallions; continue to cook for 4 minutes more or until thoroughly warmed.

Nutrition:

142 Calories

11.4g Fat

2.9g Protein

1.3g Fiber

Tofu Stuffed Zucchini

Preparation Time: 20 minutes

Cooking Time: 50 minutes

Serving: 4

Ingredients:

- 4 zucchinis, cut into halves lengthwise and scoop out the pulp
- 6 ounces firm tofu, drained and crumbled
- 2 garlic cloves, pressed
- 1/2 cup onions, chopped
- 1 tablespoon olive oil
- 1 cup tomato puree
- 1 tablespoon nutritional yeast
- 2 ounces pecans, chopped
- 1/4 teaspoon curry powder
- Sea salt and pepper, to taste

Directions:

1. In a saucepan, heat the olive oil over a moderately-high heat; cook the tofu, garlic, and onion for about 5 minutes.
2. Stir in the tomato puree and scooped zucchini pulp; add all seasonings and continue to cook for a further 5 to 6 minutes.

3. Spoon the filling into the zucchini "shells" and arrange them in a lightly greased baking dish.

4. Bake in the preheated oven at 365 degrees F for 25 to 30 minutes. Top with nutritional yeast and pecans nuts; bake for a further 5 minutes.

Nutrition:

208 Calories

14.4g Fat

6.5g Protein

4.3g Fiber

Broccoli Masala

Preparation Time: 5 minutes

Cooking Time: 15 minutes

Serving: 4

Ingredients:

- 1/4 cup sesame oil
- 1-pound broccoli florets
- 1/2 teaspoon Garam Masala
- 1 tablespoon Kasuri Methi (dried fenugreek leaves)
- 1 Badi Elaichi (black cardamom)
- 1 teaspoon garlic, pressed
- Salt and pepper, to taste

Directions:

1. Parboil the broccoli for 6 to 7 minutes until it is crisp-tender.
2. Heat the sesame oil in a wok or saucepan until sizzling. Once hot, cook your broccoli for 3 to 4 minutes. Add in the other ingredients and give it a quick stir.
3. Adjust the spices to suit your taste.

Nutrition:

100 Calories

8.2g Fat

3.7g Protein

4g Fiber

Italian-Style Tomato Crisps

Preparation Time: 10 minutes

Cooking Time: 5 hours

Serving: 6

Ingredients:

- 1 tablespoon Italian spice mix
- 1 ½ pounds Romano tomatoes, sliced
- 1/4 cup extra-virgin olive oil
- For Vegan Parmesan:
- 1/4 cup sunflower seeds
- Salt and pepper, to taste
- 1/4 teaspoon dried dill weed
- 1 teaspoon garlic powder
- 1/4 cup sesame seeds
- 1 tablespoon nutritional yeast

Directions:

1. Process all ingredients for the vegan parmesan in your food processor.
2. Toss the sliced tomatoes with the extra-virgin olive oil, Italian spice mix, and vegan parmesan.
3. Arrange the tomato slices on a parchment-lined baking sheet in a single layer. Bake at 220 degrees F about 5 hours.

Nutrition:

161 Calories

14g Fat

4.6g Protein

2.6g Fiber

Lebanese Asparagus with Baba Ghanoush

Preparation Time: 15 minutes

Cooking Time: 45 minutes

Serving: 6

Ingredients:

- 1/4 cup sesame oil
- 1 ½ pounds asparagus spears, med
- 1/2 teaspoon red pepper flakes
- Salt and pepper, to taste
- For Baba Ghanoush:
- 2 tablespoons fresh lime juice
- 2 teaspoons olive oil
- 1/2 cup onion, chopped
- 3/4-pound eggplant
- 1 teaspoon garlic, minced
- 1 tablespoon sesame paste
- 1/2 teaspoon allspice
- 1/4 teaspoon ground nutmeg
- 1/4 cup fresh parsley leaves, chopped
- Salt and ground black pepper, to taste

Directions:

1. Toss the asparagus spears with sesame oil, salt, and pepper. Arrange the asparagus spears on a foil-lined baking pan.

2. Roast in the preheated oven at 380 degrees F for 8 to 10 minutes.

3. Meanwhile, make your Baba Ghanoush. Bake eggplants in the preheated oven at 420 degrees F for 25 to 30 minutes; discard the skin and stems.

4. In a saucepan, heat 2 the olive oil over a moderately-high heat. Cook the onion and garlic until tender and fragrant; heat off.

5. Add the roasted eggplant, sautéed onion mixture, sesame paste, lime juice, and spices to your blender or food processor. Pulse until creamy and smooth.

Nutrition:

149 Calories

12.1g Fat

3.6g Protein

4.6g Fiber

Garlic Mozzarella Bread

Preparation Time: 20 minutes

Cooking Time: 65 minutes

Serving: 8

Ingredients:

- 1 cup vegan mozzarella
- 1 cup almond flour
- ½ medium onion (diced)
- 4 tbsp. ground flaxseed
- 3 tbsp. olive oil
- ½ cup water
- 1 tbsp. Italian herbs
- ½ tsp. baking powder
- 2 garlic cloves (minced)
- Optional: ¼ cup black olives

Directions:

1. Preheat the oven to 350°F/175°C and line a large loaf pan with parchment paper. In a small bowl, combine the water with the ground flaxseed. Let the flaxseed soak for about 10 minutes.

2. Put the soaked seeds in a food processor with all the other ingredients, and pulse until they are combined into a smooth batter. Scrape the

sides of the food processor if necessary. Transfer the batter onto the loaf pan and let the mixture sit for a few minutes.

3. Put the loaf pan in the oven and bake the bread for 50 minutes, until the bread is firm and browned on top. Take the loaf pan out of the oven and allow the bread to cool down completely.

4. Transfer the bread to a cutting board and slice it into 8 slices. Serve and enjoy!

5. Alternatively, store the bread in an airtight container in the fridge and consume within 4 days. Store for a maximum of 60 days in the freezer and thaw at room temperature before serving.

Nutrition:

256 Calories

23.5 g. Fat

6.6 g. Protein

Truffle Parmesan Bread

Preparation Time: 20 minutes

Cooking Time: 65 minutes

Serving: 8

Ingredients:

- 1 cup truffle parmesan cheese
- 1 cup almond flour
- ½ cup button mushrooms (diced)
- 2 tbsp. soy sauce
- ½ medium onion (finely chopped)
- ½ cup ground flaxseed
- 4 tbsp. olive oil
- ½ cup water
- 1 tsp. dried thyme
- 1 tsp. dried basil
- 1 tsp. black pepper
- ½ tsp. baking powder

Directions:

1. Preheat the oven to 350°F/175°C and line a large loaf pan with parchment paper. In a small bowl, combine the water with the ground flaxseed. Let the flaxseed soak for about 10 minutes.

2. Meanwhile, put a medium-sized frying pan over medium-high heat and add a tablespoon of olive oil. When the oil is warm, add the chopped onions, mushrooms, and soy sauce to the frying pan and stir-fry until the mushrooms and onion have softened.

3. Put the flaxseed, stir-fried ingredients, and all remaining ingredients in a food processor and pulse until all ingredients are combined into a smooth mixture. Scrape down the sides of the food processor if necessary.

4. Transfer the mixture into the loaf pan and let the mixture sit for a few minutes. Put the loaf pan in the oven and bake the bread for about 50 minutes, until the bread is firm and browned on top.

5. Take the loaf pan out of the oven and allow the bread to cool down completely. Transfer the bread to a cutting board and slice it into 8 slices. Serve warm or cold and enjoy!

6. Alternatively, store the bread in an airtight container in the fridge and consume within 4 days. Store for a maximum of 60 days in the

freezer and thaw at room temperature before serving.

Nutrition:

296 Calories

26.9 g. Fat

7.7 g. Protein

Truffle Parmesan Salad

Preparation Time: 10 minutes

Cooking Time: 15 minutes

Serving: 4

Ingredients:

- 4 cups kale (chopped)
- ½ cup truffle parmesan cheese
- 1 tsp. Dijon mustard
- 2 tbsp. olive oil
- 2 tbsp. lemon juice
- Salt and pepper to taste
- Optional: 2 tbsp. water

Directions:

1. Rinse the kale with cold water, then drain the kale and put it into a large bowl. In a medium-sized bowl, mix the remaining ingredients into a dressing. Pour the dressing over the kale and stir gently to cover the kale evenly.
2. Transfer the large bowl to the fridge and allow the salad to chill for up to one hour – doing so will guarantee a better flavor. Alternatively, the salad can be served right away. Enjoy!

3. Alternatively, store the salad in the fridge using an airtight container and consume within 2 days.

Nutrition:

199 Calories

16.6 g Fat

3.5 g. Protein

1.9 g. Fiber

Cashew Siam Salad

Preparation Time: 10 minutes

Cooking Time: 15 minutes

Serving: 4

Ingredients:

Salad:

- 4 cups baby spinach (rinsed, drained)
- ½ cup pickled red cabbage

Dressing:

- 1-inch piece ginger (finely chopped)
- 1 tsp. chili garlic paste
- 1 tbsp. soy sauce
- ½ tbsp. rice vinegar
- 1 tbsp. sesame oil
- 3 tbsp. avocado oil
- Toppings:
- ½ cup raw cashews (unsalted)
- Optional: ¼ cup fresh cilantro (chopped)

Directions:

1. Put the spinach and red cabbage in a large bowl. Toss to combine and set the salad aside. Toast the cashews in a frying pan over medium-high heat, stirring occasionally until the cashews are golden brown. This should take

about 3 minutes. Turn off the heat and set the frying pan aside.

2. Mix all the dressing ingredients in medium-sized bowl and use a spoon to mix them into a smooth dressing. Pour the dressing over the spinach salad and top with the toasted cashews.

3. Toss the salad to combine all ingredients and transfer the large bowl to the fridge. Allow the salad to chill for up to one hour – doing so will guarantee a better flavor. Alternatively, the salad can be served right away, topped with the optional cilantro. Enjoy!

4. Alternatively, store the salad in the fridge using an airtight container and consume within 2 days.

Nutrition:

236 Calories

21.6 g. Fat

4.2 g. Protein

1.3 g. Fiber

Avocado and Cauliflower Hummus

Preparation Time: 10 minutes

Cooking Time: 20 minutes

Serving: 2

Ingredients:

- 1 medium cauliflower (stem removed and chopped)
- 1 large Hass avocado (peeled, pitted, and chopped)
- ¼ cup extra virgin olive oil
- 2 garlic cloves
- ½ tbsp. lemon juice
- ½ tsp. onion powder
- Sea salt and ground black pepper to taste
- 2 large carrots (peeled and cut into fries, or use store-bought raw carrot fries)
- Optional: ¼ cup fresh cilantro (chopped)

Directions:

1. Preheat the oven to 450°F/220°C, and line a baking tray with aluminum foil. Put the chopped cauliflower on the baking tray and drizzle with 2 tablespoons of olive oil.
2. Roast the chopped cauliflower in the oven for 20-25 minutes, until lightly brown. Remove the

tray from the oven and allow the cauliflower to cool down.

3. Add all the ingredients—except the carrots and optional fresh cilantro—to a food processor or blender, and blend the ingredients into a smooth hummus. Transfer the hummus to a medium-sized bowl, cover, and put it in the fridge for at least 30 minutes.

4. Take the hummus out of the fridge and, if desired, top it with the optional chopped cilantro and more salt and pepper to taste; serve with the carrot fries, and enjoy!

5. Alternatively, store it in the fridge in an airtight container, and consume within 2 days

Nutrition:

416 Calories

40.3g. Fat

3.3g. Protein

10.3g. Fiber

Raw Zoodles with

Avocado and Nuts

Preparation Time: 5 minutes

Cooking Time: 10 minutes

Serving: 2

Ingredients:

- 1 medium zucchini (spiralized into zoodles or sliced into very thin slices)
- 1½ cups basil
- 1/3 cup water
- 5 tbsp. pine nuts
- 2 tbsp. lemon juice
- 1 medium avocado (peeled, pitted, and sliced)
- Optional: 2 tbsp. olive oil
- 6 yellow cherry tomatoes (halved)
- Optional: 6 red cherry tomatoes (halved)
- Sea salt and black pepper to taste

Directions:

1. Add the basil, water, nuts, lemon juice, avocado slices, optional olive oil (if desired), salt, and pepper to a blender. Blend the ingredients into a smooth mixture. Add more salt and pepper to taste and blend again.
2. Divide the sauce and the zucchini noodles between two medium-sized bowls for serving,

and combine in each. Top the mixtures with the halved yellow cherry tomatoes, and the optional red cherry tomatoes (if desired); serve and enjoy!

3. Alternatively, store the zoodles in the fridge using an airtight container and consume within 2 days.

Nutrition:

317 Calories

28.1 g. Fat

7.2 g. Protein

8.9 g. Fiber

Cauliflower Sushi

Preparation Time: 15 minutes

Cooking Time: 30 minutes

Serving: 4

Ingredients:

Sushi Base:

- 6 cups cauliflower florets (or 15-oz. pack cauliflower rice)
- ½ cup vegan cheese (see mozzarella recipe)
- 1 medium spring onion (diced)
- 4 nori sheets
- Sea salt and pepper to taste
- 1 tbsp. rice vinegar or sushi vinegar
- Optional: 1 medium garlic clove (minced)

Filling:

- 1 medium Hass avocado (peeled, sliced)
- ½ medium cucumber (skinned, sliced)
- 4 asparagus spears
- Optional: handful of enoki mushrooms

Directions:

1. Put the cauliflower florets in a food processor or blender. Pulse the florets into a rice-like substance. When using readymade cauliflower rice, add this to the blender. Add the vegan

cheese, spring onions, and vinegar to the food processor or blender. Top these ingredients with salt and pepper to taste, and pulse everything into a chunky mixture. Make sure not to turn the ingredients into a puree by pulsing too long.

2. Taste and add more vinegar, salt, or pepper to taste. Add the optional minced garlic clove to the blender and pulse again for a few seconds. Lay out the nori sheets and spread the cauliflower rice mixture out evenly between the sheets. Make sure to leave at least 2 inches of the top and bottom edges empty.

3. Place one or more combinations of multiple filling ingredients along the center of the spread-out rice mixture. Experiment with different ingredients per nori sheet for the best flavor. Roll up each nori sheet tightly. (Using a sushi mat will make this easier.)

4. Either serve the sushi as a nori roll, or, slice each roll up into sushi pieces. Serve right away with a small amount of wasabi, pickled ginger, and soy sauce!

5. Alternatively, store the sushi in an airtight container in the fridge and consume within 3 days. Store the sushi in the freezer for a maximum of 60 days and thaw at room temperature.

Nutrition:

189 Calories

14.4 g. Fat

6.1 g. Protein

7.45 g. Fiber

Spinach and Mashed

Tofu Salad

Preparation Time: 10 minutes

Cooking Time: 20 minutes

Serving: 4

Ingredients:

- 2 8-oz. blocks firm tofu (drained)
- 4 cups baby spinach leaves
- 4 tbsp. cashew butter
- 1½ tbsp. soy sauce
- 1-inch piece ginger (finely chopped)
- 1 tsp. red miso paste
- 2 tbsp. sesame seeds
- 1 tsp. organic orange zest
- 1 tsp. nori flakes
- Optional: 2 tbsp. water

Directions:

1. Use paper towels to absorb any excess water left in the tofu before crumbling both blocks into small pieces. In a large bowl, combine the mashed tofu with the spinach leaves.

2. Mix the remaining ingredients in another small bowl and, if desired, add the optional water for a smoother dressing. Pour this dressing over the mashed tofu and spinach leaves.

3. Transfer the bowl to the fridge and allow the salad to chill for up to one hour. Doing so will guarantee a better flavor. Or, the salad can be served right away. Enjoy!

4. Alternatively, store the spinach and mashed tofu salad in the fridge using an airtight container. Consume within 2 days.

Nutrition:

166 Calories

10.7 g. Fat

11.3 g. Protein

2.8 g. Fiber

Ketogenic Curry Almond Bread

Preparation Time: 15 minutes

Cooking Time: 30 minutes

Serving: 2

Ingredients:

- ½ cup almond flour (or coconut flour)
- ¼ cup almond milk
- ¼ cup ground flaxseed
- 2 tbsp. coconut oil
- 2 tbsp. red curry paste
- ½ tsp. salt
- ½ tsp. cane sugar (or stevia powder)
- 2 kaffir lime leaves (chopped)
- 2 tsp. dried ginger (or fresh, minced)
- Optional: ¼ cup water
- Optional: 4 tbsp. coconut flakes

Directions:

1. Line a baking sheet with parchment paper. In a medium bowl, mix the almond milk with the sugar, salt, and ground flaxseeds. Stir well and let it sit for 10 minutes. Add the flour, kaffir lime leaves, and ginger to the bowl.

2. Incorporate all ingredients using your hands or an electric mixer. Add some of the optional water to make the mixing easier. Divide the dough into two pieces and flatten these out onto the baking sheet.

3. Grease both sides of the dough with the coconut oil and apply a tablespoon of red curry paste on the top side of each flattened bread. Allow the pieces of bread to rest for an hour at room temperature.

4. Preheat the oven to 400°F / 200°C. Bake the bread for about 15 minutes, until golden brown on top. Top the breads with the optional coconut flakes. Serve and enjoy!

5. Alternatively, store the breads at room temperature or in the fridge using an airtight container and consume within 1-2 days.

Nutrition:

372 Calories

34.7 g Fat

8.3 g. Protein

9.5 g. Fiber

Egg Roll Bowl

Preparation Time: 10 minutes

Cooking Time: 15 minutes

Serving: 2

Ingredients:

- 2 7-oz. packs shirataki noodles
- 1 tbsp. coconut oil
- 1 tbsp. sesame oil
- 1 tbsp. rice vinegar
- 1 12-oz. pack extra firm tofu (drained, cubed)
- 1 red onion (diced)
- 2 garlic cloves (minced)
- 1-inch fresh ginger (finely minced)
- 4 tbsp. low sodium soy sauce
- ½ cup red pickled cabbage (chopped)
- ½ cup carrots (matchsticks or julienned)

Directions:

1. In a medium bowl, rinse the shirataki noodles with cold water, drain, and set aside. Take a large skillet and put it over medium-high heat. Add the coconut oil and sesame oil to the skillet.

2. Add the rice vinegar, tofu cubes, and onions to the skillet. Stir-fry the ingredients until the

onions start to caramelize. Blend in the garlic, ginger, and soy sauce. Allow the ingredients to cook for a minute while occasionally stirring.

3. Add the carrots to the skillet and cook for another 5 minutes while stirring occasionally. Take the skillet off the heat, divide the shirataki noodles over 2 medium bowls, top each portion with half of the tofu mixture and chopped cabbage, serve, and enjoy!

4. Alternatively, store the tofu mixture and noodles separated in the fridge. Use airtight containers and consume within 3 days. Store in the freezer for a maximum of 30 days and thaw at room temperature. Use a microwave, toaster oven or skillet to reheat the dish.

Nutrition:

269 Calories

17.6 g. Fat

16.7 g. Protein

9.4 g. Fiber

Shio Koji Karaage Tofu

Preparation Time: 10 minutes

Cooking Time: 20 minutes

Serving: 4

Ingredients:

- Extra light olive oil (for deep-frying)
- 1 12-oz. pack extra firm tofu (drained, cubed)
- 4 tbsp. Hikari Shio Koji
- 1 tsp. fresh ginger (finely chopped)
- 1 garlic clove (minced)
- 2 tsp. soy sauce
- ½ cup almond flour
- Optional: lemon wedges

Directions:

1. In a large bowl or Ziploc bag, combine the tofu cubes with the Hikari Shio Koji, ginger, garlic, and soy sauce. Use your hands to make sure the tofu is evenly coated. Cover the bowl or close the Ziploc bag and put in the fridge. Marinate the tofu for at least 30 minutes up to a maximum of 1 day.

2. Heat up a pot with enough of the olive oil to deep fry the tofu cubes. The ideal temperature for the oil is 325°F /160°F. Take the tofu cubes

out of the fridge and cover the cubes with almond flour. This can be done in the bowl or Ziploc bag. Use your hands to evenly coat all tofu cubes with flour.

3. Drop the coated cubes gently into the pot and fry until they're lightly browned. When the tofu cubes are ready, transfer them to a plate lined with paper towels to drain the excess oil.

4. Serve the shio koji karaage tofu, garnished with the optional lemon wedges if desired, and enjoy!

5. Alternatively, store the dish in an airtight container in the fridge. Consume within 3 days. Store in the freezer for a maximum of 30 days, and thaw at room temperature. Use a toaster oven or skillet to reheat the shio koji karaage tofu.

Nutrition:

355 Calories

32 g. Fat

11.3 g. Protein

Zoodle Pesto Salad

Preparation Time: 10 minutes

Cooking Time: 20 minutes

Serving: 2

Ingredients:

- 2 medium zucchinis (spiralized into zoodles or sliced lengthwise very thinly)
- ¼ cup extra virgin olive oil
- 1 ½ cups fresh baby spinach leaves
- ¼ cup walnuts (crushed)
- 1 tsp. garlic powder
- Sea salt and ground black pepper to taste
- ¼ cup capers (chopped)
- Optional: ½ cup of vegan cheese

Directions:

1. Combine all the ingredients except the zoodles, capers, and optional vegan cheese in a food processor or blender. Pulse for 1-2 minutes into a smooth pesto.
2. If desired, cook zoodles or zucchini slices for up to 4 minutes in a large skillet, with boiling water and a pinch of olive oil, over medium heat. Alternatively, the zoodles or zucchini slices can be used raw.

3. Melt the optional vegan cheese on a plate in the microwave for about 40 seconds, until it is melted and spreadable.

4. Serve the raw or cooked zoodles with the pesto, garnished with the chopped capers. Top the dish with the optional molten vegan cheese and add more salt and pepper to taste.

5. Alternatively, store the zoodle pesto salad in a multiple-compartment airtight container in the fridge and consume within 2 days. Store in the freezer for a maximum of 30 days and thaw at room temperature. Reheat without the zoodles in the microwave for up to 30 seconds.

Nutrition:

389 Calories

37 g. Fat

5.9 g. Protein

4.2 g. Fiber

Cucumber Edamame Salad

Preparation Time: 15 minutes

Cooking Time: 40 minutes

Serving: 2

Ingredients:

- 3 tbsp. avocado oil
- 1 cup cucumber (sliced into thin rounds)
- ½ cup fresh sugar snap peas (sliced or whole)
- ½ cup fresh edamame
- ¼ cup radish (sliced)
- 1 large Hass avocado (peeled, pitted, sliced)
- 1 nori sheet (crumbled)
- 2 tsp. roasted sesame seeds
- 1 tsp. salt

Directions:

1. Bring a medium-sized pot filled half way with water to a boil over medium-high heat. Add the sugar snaps and cook them for about 2 minutes. Take the pot off the heat, drain the excess water, transfer the sugar snaps to a medium-sized bowl and set aside for now.

2. Fill the pot with water again, add the teaspoon of salt and bring to a boil over medium-high heat. Add the edamame to the pot and let them

cook for about 6 minutes. Take the pot off the heat, drain the excess water, transfer the soybeans to the bowl with sugar snaps and let them cool down for about 5 minutes.

3. Combine all ingredients, except the nori crumbs and roasted sesame seeds, in a medium-sized bowl. Carefully stir, using a spoon, until all ingredients are evenly coated in oil. Top the salad with the nori crumbs and roasted sesame seeds. Transfer the bowl to the fridge and allow the salad to cool for at least 30 minutes.

4. Alternatively, store the cucumber edamame salad and the nori and sesame seeds in separate airtight containers in the fridge. Consume within 2 days. Store in the freezer for a maximum of 30 days and thaw at room temperature before serving.

Nutrition:

409 Calories

38.25 g. Fat

7.6 g. Protein

9.2 g. Fiber

Flourless Bread

Preparation Time: 10 minutes

Cooking Time: 20 minutes

Serving: 12

Ingredients:

- 1 tsp. coconut oil
- 6 tbsp. water
- 2 tbsp. flax seed (ground)
- 1 cup almond butter
- 1 cup pumpkin (pitted, diced, and cooked. Alternatively, use canned pumpkin puree.)
- 1 ½ tsp. baking powder
- ½ tsp. cinnamon
- 1 cup organic soy protein (vanilla flavor)
- ¼ cup pumpkin seeds (raw or roasted)
- Optional: ½ tsp. nutmeg

Directions:

1. Preheat the oven to 320°F/160°C. Line a large loaf pan with parchment paper and grease the paper with the coconut oil. In a small bowl, combine the water with the flax seeds. Allow the seeds to soak for about 10 minutes.
2. After 10 minutes, put all the ingredients except the roasted pumpkin seeds in a blender or food

processor. If desired, include the optional nutmeg. Pulse until ingredients are combined into a smooth batter, scraping the sides of the blender or food processor if necessary.

3. Transfer the batter into the loaf pan and allow the mixture to sit for a few minutes. Put the loaf pan in the oven and bake the bread for 20 minutes. Remove the bread and top it with the pumpkin seeds, then bake for another 15-20 minutes, or until a knife comes out clean. Take the loaf pan out of the oven and allow the bread to cool. Transfer the bread to a cutting board and slice it into 12 slices.

4. Alternatively, store the bread in an airtight container in the fridge and consume within 4 days. Store for a maximum of 60 days in the freezer and thaw at room temperature before serving.

5. Tip: Serve the bread with a vegan cheese or guacamole!

Nutrition:

191 Calories

14.7 g. Fat

10.8 g. Protein

2.9 g. Fiber

Walnut & Mushroom Loaf

Preparation Time: 4 hours

Cooking Time: 1 hour

Serving: 10

Ingredients:

- 2 tbsp. coconut oil
- 2 cups walnuts
- 3 portobello mushroom caps (stems removed)
- ½ cup green onion (sliced)
- 2 cups fresh baby spinach leaves
- Marinade:
- 1 tbsp. balsamic vinegar
- 1 tbsp. soy sauce
- 1 tsp. cumin
- Pinch of Himalayan salt

Directions:

1. Grease a large cheese mold or loaf pan that fits in a dehydrator with coconut oil and set it aside. In a medium-sized bowl, cover the walnuts with water and soak them for at least 8 hours. Rinse and drain the walnuts after soaking, and make sure no water is left.
2. Mix all the marinade ingredients in a small bowl until no lumps remain. Cut the portobello

mushroom caps into small pieces. Add to the marinade bowl and stir until all pieces are evenly coated. Set the mushrooms aside for 30 minutes.

3. After 30 minutes, put the walnuts into a food processor or blender and pulse into tiny bits. Add the marinated mushroom pieces and green onion and continue pulsing the ingredients into a smooth mixture with tiny chunks. This should take about 2 minutes.

4. Transfer the mixture into the cheese mold and sprinkle with some additional salt. Cover the mold with parchment paper and place the walnut and mushroom loaf into a dehydrator. Dehydrate the loaf at 90°F/32°C for about 2 hours.

5. After 2 hours, flip the mold upside down and dehydrate for another 2 hours. Take the loaf out of the mold and cut it into 10 slices or chunks. Serve each slice with a handful of baby spinach leaves and enjoy!

6. Alternatively, store the walnut and mushroom loaf slices in an airtight container in the fridge and consume within 3 days.

Nutrition:

195 Calories

18.25 g. Fat

4.5 g. Protein

2.1 g. Fiber

Maple Low Carb Oatmeal

Preparation Time: 5 minutes

Cooking Time: 5 minutes

Servings: 1

Ingredients:

- 1/2 cups pecans
- 1/2 cups walnuts
- 1/4 cup sunflower seeds
- 1/4 cup coconut chips
- 4 cups unsweetened almond milk
- 4 tbsp chia seeds
- 3/8 tsp stevia powder
- 1/2 tsp cinnamon
- 1 tsp maple seasoning (discretionary)

Directions:

1. Include the pecans, walnuts and sunflower seeds to a food processor and repeat a couple of times to break them up.
2. In a bowl, include all of the ingredients.
3. Put on low and stew for a decent 20-30 minutes, mixing, until the chia seeds have consumed the greater part of the fluid.

4. Remember to mix as the seeds can adhere to your pot at the base!

5. At the point when the cereal has thickened, turn off the heat and serve hot. You can likewise let it chill off and store it in the cooler for your morning meal the following day.

6. Present with new foods grown from the ground other wanted garnishes.

Nutrition:

374 Calories

34.59g Fat

182mg Sodium

12.37g Carbohydrates

Easy Curried Tofu Scramble

Preparation Time: 3 minutes

Cooking Time: 5 minutes

Servings: 1

Ingredients:

Tofu Scramble

- 2-3 tbsp low-sodium vegetable soup
- 1/2 medium onion, diced
- 1 huge red pepper, diced
- 6 oz mushrooms, cut
- 1 square firm or additional firm natural tofu, squeezed and depleted
- 2-3 cups generally hacked greens (kale, spinach, arugula, dandelion greens)

Curry Seasoning Mix

- 1/2 tsp curry powder
- 1/2 tsp garlic powder
- 1/2 tsp cumin
- 1/4 tsp coriander
- 1/4 tsp paprika
- 1/4 tsp turmeric (for shading!)
- 1/4 tsp garam masala
- 1/4 tsp dark salt (Or Himalayan pink ocean salt)

- 1 tbsp water (sufficiently just to combine the seasonings into a "sauce")

Directions:

1. In a pan of larger size, sauté the onions in vegetable soup for 5 minutes.
2. Add the cut mushrooms and diced red peppers. Cook for 10 minutes.
3. Then add the cooked veggies to the other side of the pan. Put the square of squeezed and depleted tofu on the opposite side of the skillet and split it up into pieces utilizing a wooden spatula.
4. Sauté for 2-3 minutes or until hot.
5. Put the ingredients of the seasonings into a little bowl and add simply enough water to have the option to whisk it together.
6. Pour the blend over the split-up tofu and hurl until each piece is covered. Combine the veggies and tofu.
7. Include the greens, spread the container and cook for 5 minutes or until the greens have withered. Serve hot, and top with green onions and hot sauce!

Nutrition:

119 Calories

9g Carbohydrates

11g Protein

5g Fat:

Vegan Low Carb Superfood Bowl

Preparation Time: 5 minutes

Cooking Time: 10 minutes

Servings: 1

Ingredients:

- 1 cup non-dairy milk
- 1/4 cup protein powder, see notes underneath
- 2 tbsp chia seeds
- 5 tbsp hemp seeds
- 2 tbsp unsweetened coconut pieces
- Extra Mix-ins:
- blended berries, blueberries as well as strawberries
- walnuts, chopped
- pecans, chopped

Directions:

1. Include the non-dairy milk, protein powder, chia seeds, hemp seeds, and unsweetened coconut into a container or compartment.
2. Blend/shake well so the protein powder is completely consolidated with the remainder of the ingredients.
3. Spot in the ice chest medium-term.

4. Next morning, include new or frozen blended berries and slashed nuts! Appreciate cold!

Nutrition:

500 Calories

35g Fat

20g Carbohydrates

30g Protein

Yogurt Parfait

Preparation Time: 3 minutes

Cooking Time: 5 minutes

Servings: 2

Ingredients:

- 2 tablespoons crude blended nuts chopped
- 1/4 cup new berries
- 1 two great yogurt strawberry or peach

Directions:

1. Layer chopped nuts, berries, and yogurt in a glass bowl, container or include ingredients directly into the yogurt cup. Mix thoroughly
2. Enjoy the delight!
3. Notes:
4. For toasted nuts, sprinkle with avocado oil. Hurl with a touch of ocean salt and priest natural product sugar. Heat at 325 for 8 minutes. Cool the coarsely slash.

Nutrition:

283 Calories

10g Carbohydrates

14g Protein

17g Fat

3g Fiber

Shirataki Noodles with Almond Butter Sauce

Preparation Time: 10 minutes

Cooking Time: 30 minutes

Servings: 1

Ingredients:

- 1 tbsp mellow olive oil or coconut oil
- cloves garlic, minced
- spring onions, diced
- 100 g since quite a while ago stemmed broccoli
- 1 little carrot, cut into little mallet
- 1/4 cabbage, destroyed
- 1 pack, g Shirataki noodles
- 1 tbsp almond margarine
- 1 or 2 tsp sriracha sauce, contingent upon how fiery you need it
- 2 tbsp coconut amino

Directions:

1. Warmth the olive oil in a wok or enormous pot on a medium warmth and include the garlic and onions. Cook for several minutes until mollified, at that point include the remainder of the veg.

2. While the vegetables are cooking, set up your shirataki noodles by discharging them out of

the parcel and flushing them well with warm water. Include them in with the vegetables.

3. Once everything is just about cooked, include the almond spread, sriracha and coconut amino. Mix into the vegetables and noodles to make a sauce and warm through.

4. Serve and appreciate!

Nutrition:

190 Calories

19.3g Sugars

7.9g Fiber

8.1g Protein

Chocolate Sea Salt Smoothie

Preparation Time: 5 minutes

Cooking Time: 0 minute

Servings: 2

Ingredient:

- 1 avocado (frozen or not)
- 2 cups almond milk
- 1 tbsp tahini
- ¼ cup cocoa powder
- 1 scoop perfect Ketogenic chocolate base

Directions:

1. Combine all the ingredients in a high-speed blender and mix until you get a soft smoothie. Add ice and enjoy!

Nutrition:

235 calories

20g fat

11.25 carbohydrates

Ingredient Zucchini Lasagna

Preparation Time: 10 minutes

Cooking Time: 1 hour 20 minutes

Servings: 9

Ingredient:

For ricotta

- 3 cups raw macadamia nuts or soaked blanched almonds
- 2 tbsp nutritional yeast
- 2 tsp dried oregano
- 1 tsp sea salt
- 1/2 cup water or more as needed
- 1/4 cup vegan parmesan cheese
- 1/2 cup fresh basil, chopped
- 1 medium lemon, juiced
- Black pepper to taste

Sauce:

- 1 28-oz jar favorite marinara sauce
- 3 medium zucchini squash thinly sliced

Directions:

1. Preheat the oven to 375 degrees Fahrenheit Put macadamia nuts to a food processor. Add the remaining ingredients and continue to puree the mixture. You want to create a fine paste.

2. Taste and adjust the seasonings depending on your personal preferences. Pour 1 cup of marinara sauce in a baking dish. Start creating the lasagna layers using thinly sliced zucchini

3. Scoop small amounts of ricotta mixture on the zucchini and spread it into a thin layer. Continue the layering until you've run out of zucchini or space for it. Sprinkle parmesan cheese on the topmost layer.

4. Cover the pan with foil and bake for 45 minutes. Remove the foil and bake for 15 minutes more. Allow it to cool for 15 minutes before serving. Serve immediately.

5. The lasagna will keep for 3 days in the fridge.

Nutrition:

338 calories

34g fat

10g carbohydrates

Vegan Ketogenic Scramble

Preparation Time: 10 minutes

Cooking Time: 15 minutes

Servings: 1

Ingredient:

- 14 oz. firm tofu
- 3 tbsp. avocado oil
- 2 tbsp. yellow onion, diced
  - tbsp. nutritional yeast
- ½ tsp. turmeric
- ½ tsp. garlic powder
- ½ tsp. salt
- 1 cup baby spinach
- 3 grape tomatoes
- 3 oz. vegan cheddar cheese

Directions:

1. Start by squeezing the water out of the tofu block using a clean cloth or a paper towel. Grab a skillet and put it on medium heat. Sauté the chopped onion in a small amount of avocado oil until it starts to caramelize

2. Using a potato masher, crumble the tofu on the skillet. Do this thoroughly until the tofu looks a lot like scrambled eggs. Drizzle some more of

the avocado oil onto the mix together with the dry seasonings. Stir thoroughly and evenly distribute the flavor.

3. Cook under medium heat, occasionally stirring to avoid burning of the tofu. You'd want most of the liquid to evaporate until you get a nice chunk of scrambled tofu. Fold the baby spinach, cheese, and diced tomato. Cook for a few more minutes until the cheese melted. Serve and enjoy!

Nutrition:

212 calories

17.5g of fat

10g protein

Low Carb Ramen

Preparation Time: 10 minutes

Cooking Time: 30 minutes

Servings: 4

Ingredient:

- 4 cups filtered water
- 4 pastured eggs
- 1 tbsp sugar-free red curry paste
- 1 tbsp coconut oil
- 2 tsp ground ginger
- 1 tsp ground turmeric
- 1 tsp garlic powder
- 2 cups full-fat canned coconut milk
- 1 cup of purple cabbage, chopped
- 1 cup of large-sized shredded rainbow carrots
- 1 cup Brussels sprouts, halved
- 2 large zucchinis, spiralized
- Salt and pepper to taste

Directions:

1. Grab a large pot and pour the water inside it, bringing it to a boil. When boiling, add the coconut milk and spices. Reduce the heat to medium-low. Put in the cabbage, Brussel sprouts, and carrots. Stir in a while before

adding the curry paste and coconut oil. Cook until the vegetables are soft and tender. This should take about 20 minutes

2. While waiting, soft boil the eggs. This should take about 6 minutes. Take it out of the pot and put in cold water.

3. When the vegetables are soft, put in the zucchini and allow it to cook for 4 minutes. Your vegetarian ramen is ready. Serve it with the peeled and halved eggs. Put in some lime juice and cilantro.

Nutrition:

237 calories

15g fat

15g total carbohydrates

Low Carb Smoked Salmon Chowder

Preparation Time: 10 minutes

Cooking Time: 20 minutes

Servings: 6

Ingredient:

- 1 stalk celery chopped
- 1 clove garlic minced
- 2 tbsp salted butter
- 2 tbsp capers
- 2 tbsp chopped red onion
- 1 tbsp tomato paste
- ½ tsp salt
- ¼ cup chopped onion
- 1½ cups chicken broth
- 1½ cups heavy whipping cream
- 4 oz cream cheese
- 6 oz smoked salmon hot smoked, chopped

Directions:

1. Grab a large saucepan and melt butter in it using medium heat. Put onion, celery, and sprinkle some salt onto the pan. Sauté until the vegetables are tender.

2. Put in the onion until fragrant. Add the chicken broth and tomato paste. Allow the mix to

simmer, constantly stirring   until you get a smooth concoction.

3. In the meantime, put the cream cheese in a blender and put some of the broth mixture inside it. Blend until smooth. You can do this slowly if this will make it easier. Put the broth back in the saucepan and add the salmon, capers, and cream.

4. Allow it to simmer again for a few minutes. The soup is ready now. Before serving, try sprinkling some chopped red onion on top.

Nutrition:

373 calories

31.84g carbohydrates

0.5g fiber

Ketogenic Bone Broth

Preparation Time: 10 minutes

Cooking Time: 80 minutes

Servings: 12

Ingredient:

- 3 Pastured Chicken Carcasses
- 10 cups of filtered water
- 2 tbsp. peppercorns
- 3 tsp turmeric
- 1 tsp salt
- 2 tbsp apple cider vinegar
- 1 lemon
- 3 bay leaves

Directions:

1. Preheat the oven to 400 degrees Fahrenheit. Put the bones on a sheet pan and slightly sprinkle with salt. Roast the chicken for 45 minutes.
2. Transfer the cooked chicken to the slow cooker bowl. Put in the peppercorns, apple cider vinegar, water, and bay leaves Cook on low heat for 23 hours.
3. When done, strain the bowl using a fine mesh sieve. Discard the solid ingredients. Divide the

broth in mason jars, about 2 cups each container.

4. Put in 1 tsp of turmeric for each day and 2 slices of lemon. If you're putting it in a large container, just make sure to maintain the ration. Hence, if the large container has 4 cups worth of broth, you should put 2 teaspoons of turmeric and 4 slices of lemon inside.

5. Heat slowly and serve when needed

Nutrition:

70 calories

4g fat

1g carbohydrates

Slow Cooker Vegetable Beef

Preparation Time: 10 minutes

Cooking Time: 70 minutes

Servings: 12

Ingredient:

- 4 slices bacon sliced into 1/2-inch pieces
- 2 pounds stew meat cut into 1" cubes, patted dry
- 1 small celeriac diced
- 2 tbsp red wine vinegar
- 2 tbsp tomato paste
- 1/2 tsp dried rosemary
- 1/2 tsp dried thyme
- 1/2 tsp ground black pepper
- 1 tsp sea salt
- 1/4 cup green beans cut into 1-inch pieces
- 1/4 cup carrots diced
- 1 28 oz can dice tomatoes
- 2 cloves garlic crushed
- 32 oz beef broth low-sodium
- 1 medium yellow onion chopped

Directions:

1. Put a large skillet on medium high heat. Cook bacon until crispy and store it in the fridge for later.

2. Remove most of the bacon grease, keeping only a small amount enough to cook the beef cubes in small batches. Season them with salt and pepper.

3. Cook until the beef cubes are browned. You don't have to cook the meat thoroughly, just sear it a little at the side. When brown, place the beef in a slow cooker crock.

4. Once all the beef cubes are in the slow cooker, turn your attention to the skillet. Lower the heat to medium and add vinegar to the skillet. Stir the vinegar around until you get a thicker consistency.

5. Pour ¼ cup of the broth in the skillet. When done, pour the liquid in the slow cooker.

6. Remember, we only transferred ¼ cup of the broth to the skillet. The remaining broth will now be cooked in the pan. This time, you'll beading the celeriac, carrots, diced tomatoes, tomato paste, onion, green beans, rosemary,

thyme, and salt to the mixture. Put some pepper as well depending on the taste.

7. Cook for 5 minutes before transferring the whole thin to the slow cooker as well. Stir constantly for 5 minutes.

8. Cover the slow cooker and set it to run for 7 hours. Taste every 2 hours and adjust as needed. Garnish with the bacon bits when serving.

Nutrition:

212 calories

13g fat

6g carbohydrates

Beef Cabbage

Preparation Time: 10 minutes

Cooking Time: 35 minutes

Servings: 8

Ingredient:

- 1-pound scotch fillet steak, cut into 1-inch pieces
- 1 large onion, chopped
- 1 stalk celery, chopped
- 2 large carrots, diced
- 1 small green cabbage chopped into bite-sized pieces
- 4 cloves garlic minced
- 6 cups beef stock or broth
- 3 tbsp fresh chopped parsley plus more to serve
- 2 tbsp olive oil
- 2 tsp dried thyme
- 2 tsp dried rosemary
- 2 tsp onion or garlic powder
- Salt and freshly-cracked black pepper to taste

Directions:

1. Put oil in a large pot and apply medium heat. Sear the beef on all sides until brown. They don't have to be cooked as they will be cooked

later. Put in the onions and cook them for 3 minutes

2. Put the celery and carrots. Cook them while constantly stirring for 4 minutes Put in the cabbage and continue cooking until the cabbage softens up. Put in the garlic until you get that very fragrant flavor.

3. Add the stock or broth. Follow it up with the dried herbs, parsley, and the onion or garlic powder. Remember that you're using low to medium heat all this time. Mix well and bring it to a simmer. Cover the pot with a lid and leave it like that for 15 minutes.

4. Constantly check to see if the carrots are already cooked as these will take the longest. When they're already soft, season the soup with salt and pepper to taste. Serve hot and enjoy! You can keep this in the fridge for up to 3 days or even 2 months if you freeze them.

Nutrition:

177 calories

4g carbohydrates

12g protein

Ketogenic Chicken

Preparation Time: 10 minutes

Cooking Time: 40 minutes

Servings: 4

Ingredient:

- 2 tbsp avocado oil
- 2 stalks celery, chopped
- 4 cups chicken broth
- 2 cups riced cauliflower
- 1/2 tsp dried thyme leaves
- 1/2 tsp paprika
- 1/4 cup chopped onions
- 2 cloves garlic, minced
- 1 lb. of skinless, boneless chicken thighs, cubed
- salt & pepper, to taste

Directions:

1. Start by grabbing a large saucepan and heating the oil over medium heat. Put in the onion and celery. Season it with salt and pepper before cooking. Wait until the vegetable becomes soft before adding the garlic, paprika, and thyme. You should be able to get a fragrant smell

2. Put in the broth and stir for a few minutes. Add the rice cauliflower and the chicken. Allow it to

boil before reducing it to simmer. This should take about 12 minutes or until the chicken is cooked all the way to the center. Add salt & pepper to taste

Nutrition:

196 calories

10.4g fat

1.8g fiber

www.ingramcontent.com/pod-product-compliance
Lightning Source LLC
Chambersburg PA
CBHW060959050726
47592CB00003B/1271